Contents

ideal handout to support the 1 day Emergency First Aid course EFAW and Provides an excellent resource for both trainers and candidates.

All information in this booklet is updated to the 2015 UK Resuscitation Council Guidelines. This booklet also contains public sector information published by the Health and Safety Executive and licensed under the Open Government Licence.

The information in this booklet has been compiled by an operational NHS Paramedic with over 27 years experience of providing hands on emergency treatments, and regularly delivers a range of First Aid Training Courses throughout the private, public and third sector.

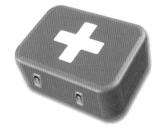

1

Key Terms

The booklet has an easy to follow layout, look out for the symbols to guide you through each medical condition.
Where there are instructions in this booklet for the emergency responder to "Call 999" it is also acceptable to "Call 112" which provides emergency assistance in all European Countries.

 Definition of Condition.

 Treatment - action to be taken.

 Signs and Symptoms to look for.

 Warning - STOP and think.

Throughout the booklet pinned post-it notes give handy hints, tips and reminders.

The Role of the First Aider

The role of the First Aider is to give help to a person who is ill or injured making sure that they are safe and comfortable until a medical professional arrives. The First Aider needs to be able to assess a situation in a systematic way (Primary/Secondary Survey) in order to ensure that the casualty, themselves and bystanders are safe, and that the situation is not made worse.

Think 3 "Ps" to remember the aims of First Aid.

P Preserve Life.

P Prevent Worsening.

P Promote Recovery.

Preventing Cross Infection
Cross infection in the first aid context is the transmitting of germs, bacteria or viruses from the casualty to the first aider or vice versa. Cross infection can occur through contact with bodily fluids, blood and potentially infectious objects or materials.

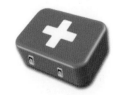

To Prevent Cross Infection

- Avoid contact with contaminated objects.
- Wash hands thoroughly.
- Wear gloves, face covering, apron and safety glasses if necessary.
- Cover any exposed cuts and grazes with waterproof plaster or similar.
- Wipe up spillages.
- Use a barrier for mouth to mouth breathing.
- Seek medical advice as soon as possible if you think you may have been contaminated by infected body fluids or blood.
- Face coverings where appropriate

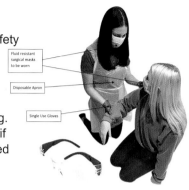

Fluid resistant surgical masks to be worn

Disposable Apron

Single Use Gloves

Recording Incidents and Accidents

In line with the Reporting of Injuries, Diseases and Dangerous Occurrences Regulations 2013 (RIDDOR) employers must report and record the following accidents and incidents in the work place:

- Work-related accidents which cause death.
- Work-related accidents which cause certain serious injuries (reportable injuries).
- Diagnosed cases of certain industrial diseases.
- Certain 'dangerous occurrences' (incidents with the potential to cause harm).

The employer should provide an Accident Book specifically for this purpose which allows the following information to be recorded:

- Time, date and location of accident/incident.
- Name, address, occupation and signature of person injured/ill.
- Description of how accident/incident happened.
- Description of injury/illness and what treatment was given.
- What happened to injured/ill following any incident.

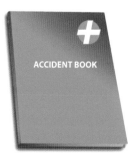

ACCIDENT BOOK

First Aid Kits

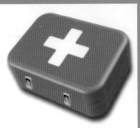

The Health and Safety (First-Aid) Regulations 1981 require employers to provide adequate and appropriate first-aid equipment, facilities and people so that employees can be given immediate help if they are injured or taken ill at work. What is 'adequate and appropriate' will depend on the type of workplace. Employers should therefore assess the first-aid needs according to the type of workplace.

It is a legal requirement that every workplace has a First Aid Kit which is a green box clearly marked with a white cross. The First Aid Kit must be easily accessible to all employees and the contents of the Kit should be checked and replenished regularly. The British Standard for First Aid Kits in the workplace is BS-8599, which recommends the contents and size of Kit required.

Size of Kit	Low Risk Workplace e.g. offices	High Risk Workplace e.g. industry
Small	Less than 25 Employees	Less than 5 Employees
Medium	25-100 Employees	5-25 Employees
Large	More than 100 Employees	More than 25 Employees

Contents	Small	Medium	Large
First Aid Guidance Notes	1	1	1
Content List	1	1	1
Nitrile Gloves	6	12	24
Face Shield	1	1	2
Foil Blanket	1	2	3
Scissors	1	1	1
Safety Pins	6	12	24
Sterile Wipes	20	30	40
Micropore Tape	1	1	1
Adhesive Waterproof Plasters	40	60	100
Medium Sterile Dressing (12cm x12 cm)	4	6	8
Large Sterile Dressing (18cm x 18cm)	1	2	2
Triangular Dressing	2	3	4
Burn Relief Dressing	1	2	2
Sterile Eye Dressing	2	3	4
Sterile Eye Wash	0	0	0
Finger Sterile Dressing	2	3	4
Conforming Bandage	1	2	2

Systematic Assessment

The Primary Survey

We need a constant intake of oxygen in order to maintain life. If this supply does not circulate our bodies and reach the brain then the brain cells will begin to die in approximately 3-4 minutes. It is therefore essential that the first priority of treatment is to ensure the casualty has a constant supply of oxygen to the blood, that the oxygenated blood is circulated throughout the body and that there is no blood loss.

The Primary Assessment/Survey is a procedure which is used to assist emergency responders in identifying immediate threats to life. The procedure prioritises the casualty's Airway, Breathing and Circulation (ABC).

A systematic way of conducting a Primary Assessment/Survey of a casualty is by using the acronym DRABC. This approach ensures that life threatening problems are first identified and that nothing is missed.

ALERT: If casualty is breathing and condition allows, carry out the secondary survey, if not breathing miss out the secondary survey and commence CPR.

Page 6

The Secondary Survey - Head to Toe Check

Once the primary survey is completed and you have responded to any life threatening injuries or conditions it is then safe to further assess the casualty. The secondary survey involves a head to toe examination checking for any other injuries or conditions in a systematic way.

Page 8

Cardiopulmonary Resuscitation – CPR

The procedure of Cardiopulmonary Resuscitation can be used if the casualty is not breathing and their heart has stopped. The technique involves a combination of chest compressions and rescue breaths to keep blood and oxygen circulating in the body.
If the casualty is not breathing firstly call 999 for an ambulance before you begin giving CPR.

Page 12

Systematic Assessment

Danger
- Make area safe for yourself, the casualty and others.
- Do not put yourself in danger or at risk.

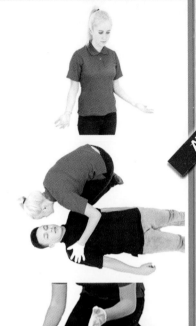

Response
- AVPU (see page opposite).
- Shake the casualty's shoulder whilst speaking loudly in both ears.
- If responsive keep the casualty in the same position, ask them what is wrong.

Airway
- Place casualty onto their back.
- Loosen any tight clothing around the neck area.
- Open the casualty's airway.
- Placing one hand on the casualty's forehead and two fingers of the other hand under their chin, gently tilt the head backward whilst lifting the chin.

Breathing
Keeping the casualty's head and chin tilted check for normal breathing by placing your ear to the casualty's cheek.

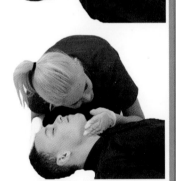

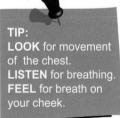

TIP:
LOOK for movement of the chest.
LISTEN for breathing.
FEEL for breath on your cheek.

Check for no longer than 10 seconds.

If the casualty is breathing normally place in recovery position and ask someone to call 999.
If the casualty is not breathing normally call 999 before starting CPR.
If there is someone near ask if there is an AED available.

AVPU Scale

Level of consciousness can be assessed using the AVPU scale:

A   **Alert**– When approached the casualty is fully alert, verbally responding to your questions and is oriented.

V   **Voice** – If no response or eye opening when spoken to, casualty responds to verbal commands but not fully alert.

P   **Pressure** – If no response to your voice, gentle shaking or tapping of the shoulders gains a response.

U   **Unresponsive** – If no response to your voice or shaking of the shoulders, the casualty is deemed as unconscious.

Unconscious Casualty

Casualties are usually considered unconscious if they cannot wake up enough to interact normally with the rescuer. The unconscious casualty loses the natural reflexes i.e. coughing and gagging.
The unconscious casualty is at risk of an obstructed airway from the tongue or vomit.

Blocked Airway

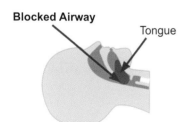

Tongue

Open Airway

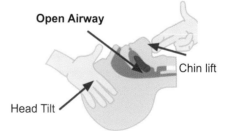

Chin lift

Head Tilt

If the casualty is unconscious consider carrying out the secondary survey (page 8) before placing the casualty into recovery position to protect the airway.

STOP A blocked airway is priority treatment and requires immediate attention.

7

Secondary Survey - Head to Toe Examination

If airway is clear and casualty is breathing normally proceed with secondary survey

History
- What happened?
- Ask the casualty or bystanders.

Signs
- Look for signs.
- What can you see or feel?

Symptoms
- What symptoms does the casualty have?
- How do they feel?

Head and Neck

Are the casualty's eyes open? Check the pupils, are they dilated, pinpoint or different sizes?

Dilated Pupils

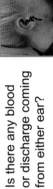

Pinpoint Pupil

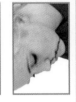

Is there any blood or discharge coming from either ear?

Is there any blood or discharge coming from the nostrils?

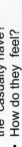

Face

What is the casualty's skin like?

- Are they paler than normal?

- Are they more flushed?

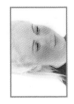

- Are their lips blue?

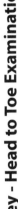

Shoulders and Chest

- Does the chest rise equally on both sides?

- Are opposite shoulders and collar bones equal?

Abdomen, Hips and Pelvis

- Are there any signs of injury?
- Is there any incontinence or bleeding?

STOP

DO NOT
PRESS ON STOMACH OR
ROCK PELVIS

Other Clues

Check:
- For medic alerts (bracelet, necklace).

- For needle marks.

- Pockets for any medication.

Limbs

- Are there any deformities or signs of fracture?
- Unusual feeling or sensations in limbs?
- Can casualty move limbs without causing pain?

Recovery Position

If the casualty is unresponsive, uninjured, breathing normally and does not need CPR, it is essential to place them in a recovery position, which ensures that their airway remains clear and open. The recovery position ensures that the tongue does not restrict the airway and prevents any vomit or fluid causing the casualty to choke.

To Place a Casualty into the Recovery Position

1. Kneel on the floor at one side of the casualty.

   Remove any glasses and straighten both legs.

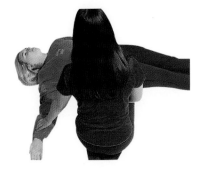

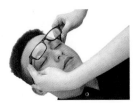

Place casualty's arm that is nearest to you out to the side with the palm upwards.

2. Bring the casualty's other hand across the body and hold the back of their hand to the side of their face.

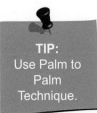

TIP:
Use Palm to Palm Technique.

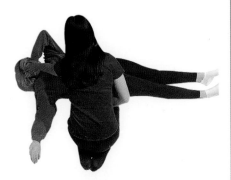

10

3. Bend the casualty's knee furthest from you to a right angle whilst keeping the foot flat on the floor.

   Maintain Palm to Palm technique.

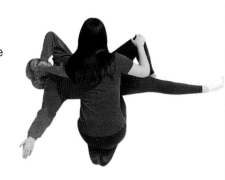

4. Roll the casualty onto their side by pulling on the knee and keeping their hand against their face.

ALERT! If the casualty is injured, only place in the recovery position if their airway is in danger i.e. vomit or blood or if being left unattended.

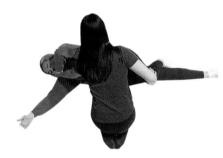

5. Place the casualty's knee at right angles with the hip, to avoid them rolling back.

   Open the casualty's airway by tilting their head back. Adjust the hand under the face to keep head tilted.

   Monitor the casualty's condition and breathing.

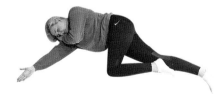

Cardiopulmonary Resuscitation – CPR

Chest Compressions and Rescue Breaths

If the casualty is not breathing you need to start CPR - chest compressions and rescue breaths keep the vital organs oxygenated.

Chest Compressions

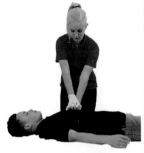

- Call 999/112 and send for a defibrillator (AED)
- Kneel down beside the casualty's chest.
- Place the heel of one hand in the centre of their chest.
- Place the heel of your other hand on top of the first hand and interlock the fingers.
- Lean over the casualty with your arms locked straight, press down on the breastbone/chest by 5-6 cm (2-2½ in).
- Release the pressure and without removing your hands allow the chest to come back up fully.
- Repeat 30 chest compressions at a rate of 100-120 strokes per minute.
- Now give 2 Rescue Breaths.

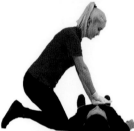

Rescue Breaths

- Open the casualty's airway using the head tilt/ chin lift technique.
- Pinch casualty's nose firmly closed.
- Take a breath and seal your lips around the casualty's mouth.
- Blow into the mouth watching the chest rise.
- Keeping airway open, remove your mouth and allow the chest to fall.
- Repeat once more.

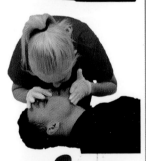

If the chest does not rise during the rescue breath:

- Check there is no obstruction in the casualty's mouth.
- Check the head tilt and chin lift are sufficient to provide a clear airway.

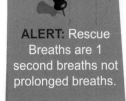

ALERT: Rescue Breaths are 1 second breaths not prolonged breaths.

Cardiopulmonary Resuscitation – CPR

Continue a cycle of giving 30 chest compressions followed by 2 rescue breaths until help arrives or the casualty shows signs of breathing normally.

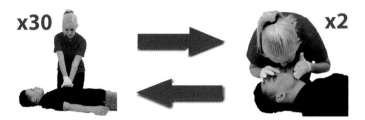

x30   **x2**

If the casualty starts breathing normally again, stop CPR and put them in the recovery position.

Carrying out CPR can be very tiring so if there is more than one emergency responder they should take over every two minutes.

For covid CPR guidelines, go to page 44

Regurgitation during CPR

Regurgitation or vomiting of gastric content is common during resuscitation. This can be caused by the pressure of the compressions causing the casualty to vomit or it may be a symptom of a cardiac condition.

Signs of Regurgitation

Vomit in mouth or gurgling sounds from the throat.
This may not be noticed until rescue breaths are being given.

Treating a Regurgitating Casualty

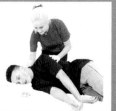

If the casualty has vomited, they should be turned onto their side with head tipped back to allow the vomit to drain out. The face can then be cleaned before rescue breaths are continued using a protective face shield.

CPR for Babies and Children

When responding to a child or baby who is not breathing normally and is unresponsive, the emergency responder can use the adult sequence of resuscitation as described earlier. Research has shown that often children do not receive resuscitation as rescuers fear causing harm. However, it is better to perform adult resuscitation on a child than to do nothing.

Administering CPR for Babies and Children

For a child or baby who is not breathing normally and is unresponsive the emergency responder can use the adult sequence of resuscitation with the following variations:

- Start with 5 initial rescue breaths before beginning compressions.
- Continue the cycle of 30 compressions to 2 breaths.
- Perform resuscitation for 1 minute before going for help.

Compressions

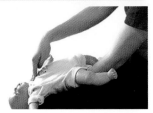

Baby under 1 year, use two fingers.

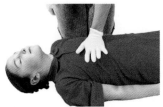

Children between 1 year and 18 years old. use one or two hands but ensure the chest is depressed at least a third of its depth.

Untrained Emergency Responder

If the emergency responder has not been trained in CPR then they can do chest compressions only (Hands Only) CPR. This will ensure that any residual oxygen in the blood stream is kept circulating.

The chest compressions should be performed at a rate of 100-120 chest compressions a minute until help arrives. If there is more than one emergency responder then they should change over every few minutes to avoid tiredness ensuring that there is minimum delay during change over.

Good Hygiene During CPR

It is essential to use good hygiene procedures during CPR in order to avoid any cross infection.

Good Hygiene Procedures

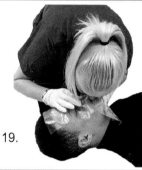

- If available use a face shield or pocket mask.
- Wear protective gloves and wash hands after.

If you are in doubt about the risk of cross infection then give 'Hands Only' CPR.

Face shields will not fully protect you from COVID 19.

Hands Only CPR

There will be occasions when you may decide not to carry out rescue breaths, e.g. you are physically unable to, chest compression only resuscitation should then be commenced.

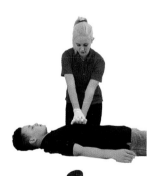

- Compression rate will be the same as above 100-120 per minute.
- If you are in any doubt as to whether the casualty has started breathing again, carry out a 10 second breathing check.
- If not breathing, continue with chest compressions.

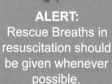

ALERT:
Rescue Breaths in resuscitation should be given whenever possible.

- To prevent fatigue, ask another rescuer to assist, changing every 2 minutes.
- CPR on a bed. if unable to lower to the floor, remove pillow, kneel on the bed to compress the mattress. compression depth needs to be increased to allow for the mattress

Automated External Defibrillator (AED)

When an AED arrives by the patients side

An AED can be safely used by an untrained responder. Additional AED training will however improve skill level and outcome.

Most AEDs will automatically switch on when the lid is opened; otherwise you will have to press the ON button.

CPR should be continued whilst the AED operator prepares the patient and equipment.

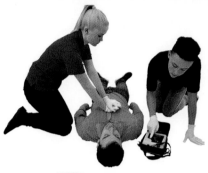

1 Set up AED.

STOP
DO NOT stop CPR at this stage.

Now follow the verbal instructions from the AED:

Attaching the Pads

- Dry chest if wet with towel or similar.
- Shave excess body hair with razor provided in kit if required. Do not delay pad placement if razor is not available.
- Remove pads from sealed packet.
- Attach the lead to the AED if not already attached.
- Remove backing from one of the pads and place below the casualty's right collar bone.
- Repeat with the second pad placing the pad around the left side over the ribs and below the nipple line.

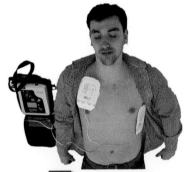

2 Attach the Pads

ALERT: Pads will work either way around.

Shock indicated – the AED will prompt you!

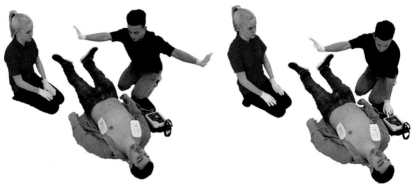

3 Nobody to touch the casualty. Announce "Stand Clear."

4 Push the flashing shock button (some AEDs will automatically deliver the shock).

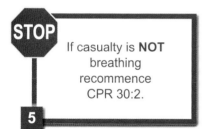

STOP
If casualty is **NOT** breathing recommence CPR 30:2.

5

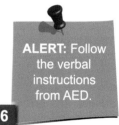

ALERT: Follow the verbal instructions from AED.

6

NO Shock indicated – the AED will prompt you!

Follow Steps 5 and 6 above:
- Recommence CPR 30:2 - Step 5.
- Follow verbal instructions from AED - Step 6.

If patient starts breathing normally:
- Place in the recovery position.
- Monitor casualty closely.
- Leave pads on casualty.

17

Emergency Response Flowchart

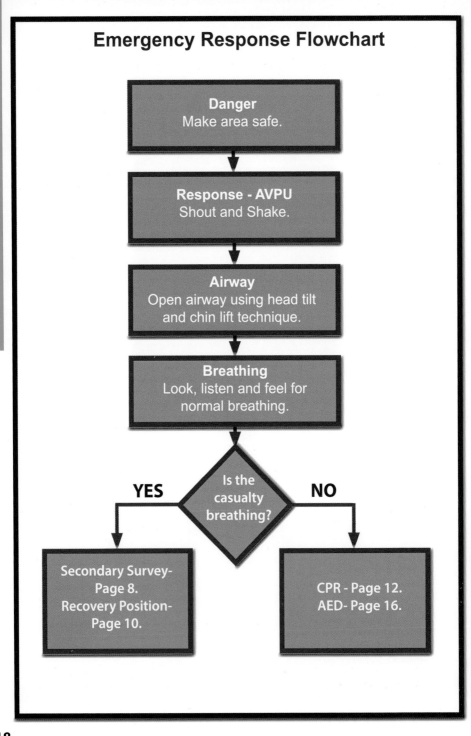

Danger
Make area safe.

Response - AVPU
Shout and Shake.

Airway
Open airway using head tilt and chin lift technique.

Breathing
Look, listen and feel for normal breathing.

Is the casualty breathing?

YES

NO

Secondary Survey-
Page 8.
Recovery Position-
Page 10.

CPR - Page 12.
AED- Page 16.

Choking

Choking occurs when a person's airway is blocked either partially or completely particularly after eating. If it is a partial obstruction they will be able to breathe, speak and cough and they should be able to clear the obstruction by coughing. If it is a complete obstruction they will be unable to breathe, speak or cough and without help they will eventually lose consciousness.

Choking Adult - Treatment

1. **Encourage the casualty to cough** If still choking, carry out back blows and abdominal thrusts. Shout for someone to call 999/112 or use a speaker phone whilst providing treatment.

2. **Back Blows**
   - Call for help.
   - Bend the casualty forward and support chest.
   - Give 5 sharp blows between the shoulder blades using the heel of your hand.
   - Check after each blow to see if obstruction has cleared.
   - If obstruction has not cleared after 5 blows move to stage 3 – Abdominal Thrusts.

3. **Abdominal Thrusts**
   - Standing behind the casualty, place your arms above the belly button and the below their ribs.
   - Link your hands by making a fist with one hand, placing the fist to the casualty's abdomen and grasping the fist with your other hand.
   - Pull sharply towards you and upwards.
   - Do this 5 times checking after each thrust to see if obstruction has cleared.

4. **Repeat**
   - Continue repeating stage 2 and 3.
   - If obstruction is not clearing call 999 whilst continuing treatment.

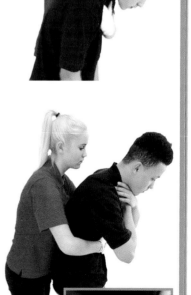

1. Encourage the child to cough.

2. Back Blows
- Call for help but don't leave the child.
- Bend the child forward or lean them over your knee.
- Give 5 sharp blows between the shoulder blades using the palm of your hand.
- Check after each blow to see if obstruction has cleared.
- If obstruction not cleared after 5 blows move to stage 3 – Abdominal Thrusts.

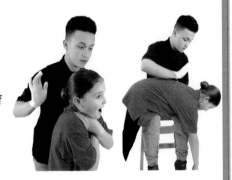

3. Abdominal Thrusts
- Standing or kneeling behind the child, place your arms around their upper abdomen between the belly button and under the ribs.
- Link your hands by making a fist with one hand, placing the fist to the casualty's abdomen and grasping the fist with your other hand.
- Pull sharply towards you and upwards.
- Do this 5 times checking after each thrust to see if obstruction has cleared.

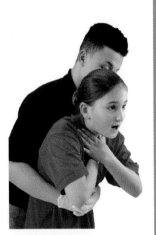

4. Repeat
- Continue repeating stage 2 and 3.
- If obstruction is not clearing call 999 whilst continuing treatment.

Unconscious Casualty
If the casualty becomes unconscious:
- Lower to the ground.
- Call 999.
- Start giving CPR 30:2.
- Continue giving CPR until they start breathing normal or help arrives.

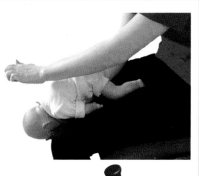

1. **Back Blows**
   - Call for help but don't leave the baby.
   - Lay baby face down over your fore-arm with their head lower than their chest.
   - Give 5 blows between the shoulder blades using heel of free hand.
   - Check after each blow to see if obstruction has cleared.
   - If obstruction has not cleared after 5 blows move to stage 2 – Chest Thrusts.

2. **Chest Thrusts**
   - Lay the baby face up across your thighs with their head lower than the chest.
   - Locate the breastbone and with two fingers give 5 thrusts compressing the chest by about a third.
   - Check between each thrust to see if the obstruction has cleared.

3. **Repeat**
   - Repeat steps 1 and 2.
   - If treatment is in ineffective call 999.
   - STOP back blows and thrusts immediately if obstruction is cleared.

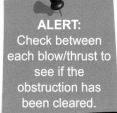

ALERT: Check between each blow/thrust to see if the obstruction has been cleared.

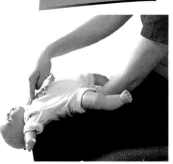

STOP

Unconscious Casualty
If the casualty becomes unconscious:
- Lower to the ground.
- Call 999.
- Start giving CPR with 30 chest compressions.
- Continue giving CPR until they start breathing normally or medical help arrives.

ALERT: If abdominal thrusts have been used on a casualty, then they should be advised to seek a medical assessment in case any injuries have been caused.

Choking

Bleeding

The circulatory system is made up of the heart, blood and blood vessels. The main role of the circulatory system is to service the body's cells with oxygen and nutrients.

Any bleeding means that there is a loss of blood from the circulatory system. The body can cope with a small amount of blood loss however, if this increases to a loss of 1/3 of the blood supply then the blood pressure will fall and the blood supply to the brain will fail which can result in death.

The treatment for severe bleeding is therefore critical to reduce the loss of blood until emergency medical help arrives.

Internal Bleeding

Internal bleeding takes place within the body and can range from minor bruising to massive bleeding. E.g. Chest, abdomen, pelvis or upper leg. This bleeding can be life threatening and medical advice should be sought immediately.

Shock developing quickly with no evident causes may mean that there is internal bleeding.

Signs of Internal Bleeding

- Chest - coughing up blood and bruising to chest wall.
- Abdomen - bruising or swelling to abdomen.
- Pelvis - bruising or swelling.
- Pale and clammy skin.
- Increased heart rate.

External Bleeding - Treatment

External bleeding can range from superficial cuts and grazes to deep wounds and amputations.

The Acronym STEP can help with remembering how to treat bleeding.

 Sit or Lay the casualty down.

 Think gloves.

 Examine the wound for foreign objects.

 Pressure: Apply continuous direct pressure over the wound for 10 minutes.

ALERT: Wear protective gloves when treating any bleeding injury.

Dressing Wounds

- Always wear gloves when dealing with wounds.
- To prevent infection a wound needs to be dressed with a sterile dressing which is slightly larger than the wound.
- The dressing should be applied firmly to control any further bleeding.
- If the blood comes through the dressing then apply a second dressing.
- If this does not work remove both dressings and start again.
- Pressure – you may need to pressure directly into the wound.

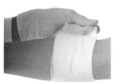

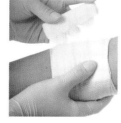

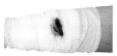

TIP: For Head Dressings, position the dressing under the natural curve at back of head to avoid it slipping up.

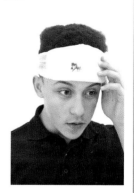

Haemostatic Agents

Haemostatic Agents or Dressings are used to stem blood flow and speed up blood clotting. Haemostatic dressings are used for life threatening bleeding where direct pressure has failed.

Use of Haemostatic Agents

1 Soak up excess blood with normal dressing.

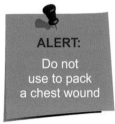

ALERT:
Do not
use to pack
a chest wound

2 Pack gauze dressing into the wound with fingers (as shown)

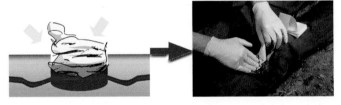

3 Apply direct pressure over the inserted gauze (as shown). Maintain pressure for up to 3 minutes.

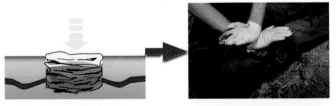

4 Cover with normal dressing and secure.

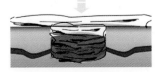

ALERT: Show empty package to medical personnel.

Images shown with permission of Celox

Tourniquets

Tourniquets provide an effective means to stopping catastrophic limb bleeding. Tourniquets are commonly used by the military worldwide and UK Emergency Services.

Inappropriate use of tourniquets, can result in nerve damage, tissue death and blood clots. Tourniquets should only be applied where the basic wound management has failed and the bleeding is life threatening.

STOP WARNING: **A tourniquet should only be used by those with relevant training.**

Use of Tourniquets

STOP Note the time of application
Call 999 Immediately.

How to apply:
- Apply to a single bone limb on upper arm or thigh, even if wound is below knee or elbow.

- If wound is on upper arm or thigh place tourniquet 5-7 cm above the wound but not over the joint.

- Tighten the strap around the limb.

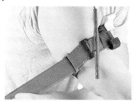

- Twist the plastic rod until the bleeding can be controlled with direct pressure.

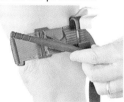

- Place the rod inside the clip locking it into place.

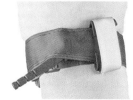

- If bleeding is not controlled consider further tightening.
- If necessary, apply a second tourniquet above the first one.
- Do not release the tourniquet, only HCP's can do this!

Amputations Treatment

- Treat the casualty for bleeding as described in STEP (page 23).
- Call 999.
- Dress the wound with a pressure dressing.
- Place the amputated limb/digit in a plastic bag or cover with cling film.
- Put the limb/digit on a bag of ice or in iced water.

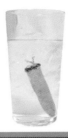

ALERT: DO NOT let the amputated limb come in direct contact with ice or water.

Embedded Objects Treatment

- Do not remove an object embedded in a wound as you could cause more harm and increased bleeding.
- Control bleeding by pressing firmly around the object.
- Dress the wound by placing dressings to the edge of the wound and not over the embedded object.

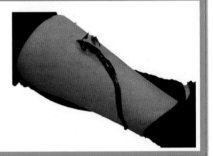

Splinters Treatment

- Clean the area with warm soapy water.
- Use a pair of sterile tweezers, to grip the splinter as close to the skin as possible and pull the splinter out.
- Squeeze the wound gently to allow it to bleed, this will help to wash out any germs.
- Wash the wound again, pat dry and cover with a dressing.
- If a splinter is embedded deeply, on a joint or difficult to remove seek further advice.

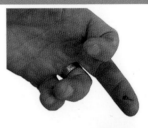

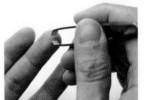

Nosebleed

Nosebleeds can occur due to the small blood vessels in the nose rupturing. Most nosebleeds only last a few minutes but they can be dangerous if there is a lot of blood loss.

If a casualty has had a blow to the head a nosebleed may suggest that their skull is fractured. This is very serious and the emergency responder should immediately call 999.

Nosebleed Treatment

If a casualty presents with a nosebleed the priority is to stop bleeding and keep airway clear.

- Sit the casualty down not lie down.
- Lean casualty forward to avoid swallowing the blood.
- Ask casualty to breathe through their mouth.

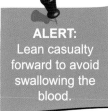

ALERT:
Lean casualty forward to avoid swallowing the blood.

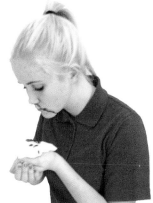

- Pinch the soft part of the casualty's nose keeping pressure for 10 minutes.
- Check every 10 minutes to see if bleeding has stopped.
- Encourage casualty not to breathe through the nose or blow their nose for a few hours.
- If the bleeding is severe, or if it lasts more than 30 minutes, or the casualty is taking anti-coagulant medication take them to hospital.

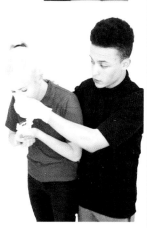

Eye Injury

Small particles of dirt or dust or a loose eyelash often land on the surface of the eye. These can be washed out of the eye with cold tap water ensuring that the water runs away from the eye.
Sharp fragments like grit, glass or metal may cause serious damage to the eye

Eye Injury Treatment

Sharp fragments like grit, glass or metal may cause serious damage to the eye.

- Place a soft sterile dressing over the eye.
- Tell casualty to keep both eyes closed to reduce any eye movement.
- Take the casualty to hospital.

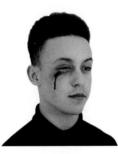 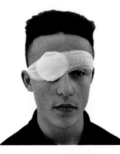

TIP: Position the dressing under the natural curve at back of head to avoid slipping.

Chemicals in the eye must be removed with copious amounts of water for 10-20 minutes.

- Wear protective gloves.
- Gently open the eye to allow water to enter.
- Ensure water runs away from clean eye.

TIP: Ask casualty to cover their non-contaminated eye with their hand.

Take casualty to hospital if there is:

- Persistent or severe eye pain.
- Foreign bodies that can't be washed out.
- Blood visible in the eye.
- An irregularly shaped pupil.
- Pain when exposed to bright light.
- Deep cuts around the eye.

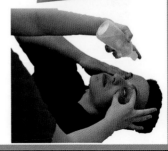

Shock

Shock is a life threatening condition which occurs when a casualty has a lack of oxygen circulating to the cells and tissues of the body Shock is caused by any injury or condition that reduces the blood supply or circulation including:
- Severe bleeding.
- Heart failure.
- Loss of body fluids such as vomiting, diarrhoea or burns.
- Severe allergic reactions.

Signs of Shock

There are key signs to look for and recognise if a casualty is experiencing shock:
- Pale, cold and clammy skin.
- Fast and shallow breathing.
- Fast and weak pulse.
- Dizziness or feeling faint.

Shock Treatment

- Treat the cause of the shock.
- Lay casualty down elevating the legs to increase the blood flow to the head.
- Call 999.
- Keep the casualty warm, cover with a blanket or coat.
- Continue checking their breathing and level of response.
- Do not give the casualty anything to eat or drink.

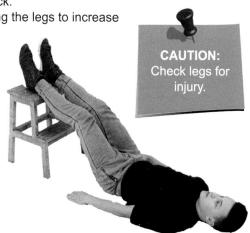

CAUTION: Check legs for injury.

Anaphylaxis

An anaphylaxis is a Severe life threatening reaction, with a rapid onset and obvious worsening of symptoms. It occurs when a person is exposed to a substance they are allergic to. The most common triggers are:
- Foods – seafood, nuts, eggs, milk or bananas.
- Insect stings.
- Medications – antibiotics, non-steroid anti inflammatory drugs.

Signs of Anaphylaxis

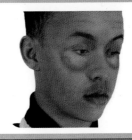

- Swollen eyes, lips, hands and feet.
- Swollen mouth, tongue or throat causing difficulty in swallowing, breathing or talking.
- Itchy, blotchy skin rash.
- Asthma symptoms, wheezy chest sounds.
- Stomach pain, nausea and vomiting.
- Dizziness or faint.
- Symptoms of shock.

Anaphylaxis Treatment

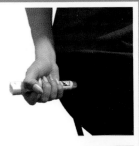

- Call 999.
- Lay the casualty down and elevate legs if they are feeling faint or dizzy.
- If breathing is difficult and not feeling faint, the casualty may be more comfortable sitting.
- If the casualty has an adrenaline auto-injector device assist casualty to administer the injection.
- Upper outside of thigh is the preferred site for auto-injecting.
- Hold in place for 10 seconds and massage the area increasing absorption.
- If casualty loses consciousness check Airway and Breathing and begin CPR if necessary.
- If a second adrenaline auto-injector is available a further dose can be given after 5 minutes if there is no improvement of symptoms.

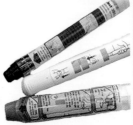

 Trained persons can administer the auto-injector if the casualty is unable to and gives consent.

Poisoning

Poisoning is caused by swallowing, injecting, inhaling, or being exposed to a harmful substance.
There are 2 types of poison:
Corrosive – acids, ammonia, bleach, petrol, turpentine, insecticides, household detergents etc.
Non- Corrosive - tablets, drugs, plants, fungi, alcohol etc.

Symptoms of Poisoning

- Abdominal pain.
- Chest pain.
- Difficulty breathing or shortness of breath, coughing.
- Dizziness or Drowsiness.
- Headache.
- Nausea and vomiting.
- Skin rash or burns.
- Unconsciousness.

STOP **DO NOT** make the casualty vomit as the vomit could block the air way.

Poisoning Treatment

Corrosive Substance Poisoning

- Ensure that the area is safe, do not endanger yourself.
- Call 999.
- If substance is on skin wash away with water.
- If swallowed, rinse the mouth and give sips of milk or water.

Non-Corrosive Substance Poisoning

- Call 999 immediately.
- Monitor casualty's airway and breathing.

Burns Treatment

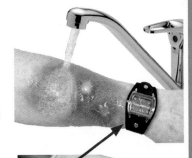

Step 1
Stop the burning by removing the source of the burn.

TIP: Cool over clothing that has stuck to the skin.

Step 2
Pour cool water onto the burn for at least twenty minutes.

TIP: Remove any jewellery.

Step 3
Remove any clothing (unless stuck to the skin) or jewellery.

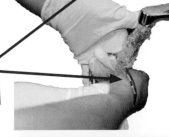

Step 4
Dress the burn, make sure the dressing isn't made of a fluffy material. Cling film is ideal for dressing a burn. Lay the cling film over the burn in layers rather than wrapping tightly around the limb as this could cut off the circulation.

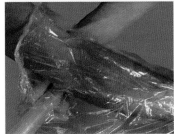

Seek Medical advice if:

- The burn is deep or charred.
- The patient is a child.
- It is an electrical or chemical burn.
- The burn affects the hands, feet, face or genitalia.
- The burn goes around a limb.
- You are unsure.

STOP

DO NOT
- Burst blisters.
- Touch the burn.
- Use fats, lotions or ointments.
- Remove anything stuck to the burn.
- Use adhesive dressings or tapes.

Heart Attack

A heart attack happens when the blood vessels supplying the heart muscle become blocked depriving the muscle of blood and oxygen, which can result in death of the heart muscle.

Signs of Heart Attack

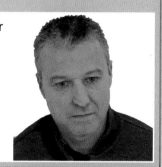

- Chest pain described as a pressure, tightness or band around the chest.
- Pain spreading from chest to both arms (most often the left arm), less common symptoms are pain in neck, back, jaw and abdomen.
- Nausea or vomiting.
- Sweating.
- Pale, cold and clammy skin.
- Dizziness.

Heart Attack Treatment

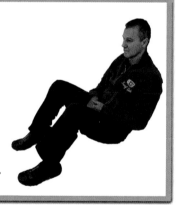

- Call 999 immediately.
- Sit the casualty down preferably on the floor with back leaning against a wall and the knees bent.
- If casualty has angina help them take their medication (See Angina below).
- Reassure the casualty and keep them calm.
- Monitor the casualty's pulse and breathing.
- If the casualty is not allergic to aspirin give them an aspirin to chew slowly. **Up to 300mg.** (See below *).

Angina

Narrowing of the blood vessels supplying the heart. When the heart is placed under demand (e.g. stress, exertion or exercise) adequate amounts of blood and oxygen fail to reach the muscle, resulting in chest pain. The patient may have medication to spray under the tongue.

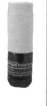

*Information: Aspirin reduces the ability of blood cells sticking and causing a blood clot.

33

Stroke

A stroke happens when the normal blood flow to the brain is blocked or when there is bleeding into the brain from a ruptured blood vessel.

A stroke is a medical emergency and can happen at any age. Part of the brain will die so it is important to get medical treatment urgently in order to ascertain the type and cause of the stroke and provide the appropriate treatment to reduce further damage to the brain.

The FAST test should be used to assist with the recognition of a stroke.

The FAST test for Stroke recognition

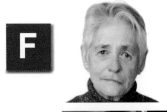

F — **FACE** - Is there facial weakness? Can the person smile? Has the face, mouth or eye drooped?

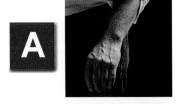

A — **ARM** - Is there a weakness in the arms? Can the person raise both arms?

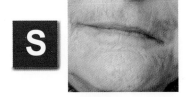

S — **SPEECH** - Is the person speaking clearly? Does the person understand what you say?

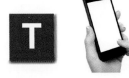

T — **Time** to call 999. If the casualty shows any one of the above signs call 999 immediately.

Further Signs and Symptoms of Stroke.

Further signs and symptoms of a stroke include:
- Numbness to one side of the body particularly the face.
- Difficulties with balance, walking or dizziness
- Coordination difficulties.
- Sudden severe headaches.
- Being suddenly confused.
- Slight problem in one or both eyes, i.e. loss of vision
- Unequal pupil sizes.

Stroke Treatment

Conscious Casualty

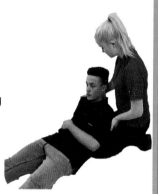

- Call 999.
- Reassure and keep casualty calm.
- If casualty is conscious lay them down keeping head and shoulders raised.
- Monitor breathing and response.

Unconscious Casualty

- Call 999.
- Place in recovery position.
- Maintain the casualty's airway and breathing.

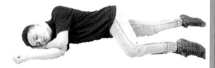

STOP

Monitor the casualty for signs of vomiting.

Types of Fractures / Broken Bones

Closed - clean break in the bone.

Open - the bone has come through the skin or is just under the surface of the skin.

Green stick - incomplete fracture in which the bone is bent. This type occurs most often in children.

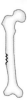

Signs and Symptoms of a Fracture

- Pain and tenderness.
- Swelling.
- Weakness and loss of strength.
- Limb may look deformed or abnormally bent.
- Movement is difficult or abnormal.
- Grinding feeling and noise on movement.

Fracture Treatment

- Support limb and keep as still as possible.
- Keep casualty warm. If immobile, the casual can get cold very quickly.
- Control any bleeding with a sterile dressing.
- Call 999 if:
  - There is a spinal, neck or head injury.
  - The casualty is finding breathing difficult.
  - There is abnormality or deformity.
  - The bone is protruding through the skin.
  - The casualty's pain is too severe to move.

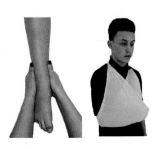

Spinal Injuries

If a casualty has a spinal bone injury there is potential for the spinal cord being damaged which may result in lack of feeling or paralysis. It is therefore essential to limit any movement and prevent any further damage.

Common causes of spinal injury:
- Severe blow to head, neck or back.
- Road traffic accident.
- Falling from a horse, cycle, etc.
- Falling from a height.
- Diving into a shallow pool.
- Collapsed rugby scrum.

STOP **DO NOT** move the casualty unless there is immediate danger.

Spinal Injury Treatment

Conscious Casualty

- Instruct casualty not to move unless they are in danger.
- If the casualty is in a car, encourage to remove themselves.
- Using your hands keep the head and neck supported in a straight line with the upper body.

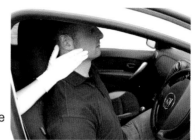

Unconscious Casualty

Airway not in danger:
- If breathing is normal this should indicate that the airway is clear.
- Keep the head and neck supported in a straight line with the upper body.
- Keep casualty warm monitoring their breathing until help arrives.

Airway in danger:
- If casualty is not breathing normally, open the airway by gently lifting the chin but avoid tilting the neck.

ALERT: If the casualty is not breathing and has a suspected spinal injury, resuscitation /CPR is the priority treatment.

If the casualty begins to vomit or the airway cannot be maintained:

Single Responder - Place in recovery position supporting head and neck as best as possible.

Assistance Available - roll the casualty onto their side keeping head and neck in line with the upper body and spine as you turn the casualty.

Epilepsy / Seizures

A seizure is caused by abnormal electrical activity in the brain and results in involuntary movement in the muscles of the arms and legs and usually causes a loss of consciousness.

Seizures are a common symptom of epilepsy but there can be other causes such as head injuries, lack of oxygen to the brain or a high body temperature (particularly in young children).

Seizure Phase

- Stiffening of arm and leg muscles.
- Groaning noise or crying out.
- Loss of consciousness and will drop to the floor.
- Blood stained saliva.
- Blue or purple lips.
- The arms and legs begin to jerk.
- The teeth may clench.
- Loss of bladder or bowel control.

Recovery Phase

- Consciousness is regained but casualty can be very sleepy.
- This stage can last for a few hours.
- The casualty can present as confused and agitated.

Seizure Treatment

- Ensure casualty is kept safe.
- Protect the casualty's head with a cushion or similar.
- Loosen any tight clothing around the neck.
- Record how long the seizure lasts.
- When seizure has stopped check Airway and Breathing.
- Place casualty in recovery position.
- Call 999 if you cannot wake them within 5 minutes, **or** if the seizure lasts longer than 5 minutes, or if you have any concerns.

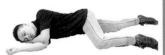

STOP

DO NOT
- Place anything in the mouth.
- Try to restrain the casualty.
- Move the casualty.

Diabetes

Diabetes is a lifelong condition where the body does not produce enough insulin to control sugar levels in the blood.

Insulin is produced by the pancreas (a gland behind the stomach). A lack of insulin means that the body is unable to burn off the sugars in the food we eat. Resulting in raised levels of sugar in the bloodstream.

People who have diabetes can sometimes have a diabetic emergency, where the sugar in their blood stream becomes too low (Hypoglycaemia).

Hypoglycaemia / Low Blood Sugar - Signs & Symptoms

- Feeling of hunger.
- Sudden onset with rapidly worsening level of response.
- Confusion, irrational behaviour.
- Shakiness and weakness.
- Pale, sweating, cold, clammy skin.
- Loss of consciousness if left untreated.

ALERT: Symptoms typically come on quickly

Hypoglycaemia / Low Blood Sugar - Treatment

Conscious Casualty

- Help the casualty to take a sugary drink or something sweet.
- If they have their own glucose gel help them to take it.
- If the casualty responds quickly, give them more to eat or drink.
- Let the casualty rest and stay with casualty until their level of response is normal and they have fully recovered.
- If their condition does not improve within 10 minutes, Call 999!

Unconscious Casualty

If casualty becomes unconscious:
- Airway, breathing check.
- Place in recovery position.
- Call 999!

ALERT: Do not try to administer a drink or food to an unconscious casualty.

Other Conditions

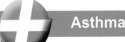

Asthma

Asthma is a common long-term condition that can cause coughing, wheezing, chest tightness and breathlessness.

Asthma is caused by inflammation of the small tubes, called bronchi, which carry air in and out of the lungs. If you have asthma, the bronchi will be inflamed and more sensitive than normal.

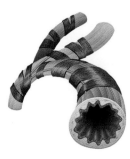
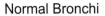
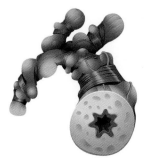

Normal Bronchi   Asthmatic Bronchi

When you come into contact with something that irritates your lungs, known as a trigger, your airways become narrow, the muscles around them tighten, and there is an increase in the production of sticky mucus (phlegm).

Generally asthma sufferers carry medication in the form of a inhaler. The inhaler sprays the medication into the mouth and is inhaled into the lungs causing the small tubes to relax and breathing to return to normal.

Asthma - Signs & Symptoms

- Shortening of breath.
- Wheezing sound when you breathe or cough.
- A tight chest – which may feel like a band is tightening around it.
- Difficulty speaking, can't complete a sentence.
- Blue lips.

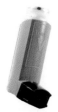

Position

Get casualty to sit upright and lean forward to assist breathing.

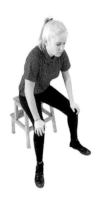

ALERT: If the casualty doesn't have their medication with them Call 999.

Medication

Encourage the casualty to take one puff of their inhaler every 30-60 seconds for up to 10 puffs, repeating if they do not feel better after a few minutes. If the casualty has difficulty using the inhaler, if available a spacer device can be used.

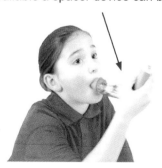

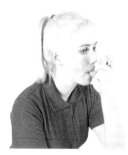

If the attack is severe and the casualty does not seem to be improving then call 999 for emergency help.

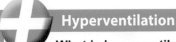

Hyperventilation

What is hyperventilation syndrome?

Hyperventilation syndrome happens when we over-breathe. This causes a decrease in the carbon dioxide levels in the lungs and blood.

Signs & Symptoms

- Unnaturally deep, rapid breathing.
- Cramps in the hands and feet.
- Flushed skin.
- Dizziness, faint.

Hyperventilation Treatment

- Reassure the casualty but be firm.
- Explain to them that they are hyperventilating.
- Coach their breathing, tell them to count slowly.
- Call 999 if you cant get them to control their breathing.

STOP DO NOT use a paper bag to control their breathing.

Insect Bites / Stings.

Insect stings from a bee, wasp or hornet can be painful but are usually not dangerous. First there is a sharp pain, followed by mild swelling, redness and soreness.

Sometimes they can cause the body to have a severe allergic reaction (anaphylactic shock), so it's important to look out for this and get medical help quickly if necessary.

Signs of Insect Bites / Stings

The main signs to look for with insect bites or stings are:
- A sting or burning pain at the site.
- Redness which and may even spread several centimetres around the sting.
- Swelling that may spread across the site and even to the whole limb.
- Itchiness at the site.

Treatment for Insect Bites / Stings

- If you can see the sting, brush or scrape it off sideways.
- Place an ice pack or a cold flannel over the wound to reduce the swelling.
- Elevate the area to reduce swelling.
- If the sting is in the mouth or throat give the casualty an ice cube to suck or some cold water to sip.
- Monitor the casualty's breathing, pulse and level of response.
- If you notice any signs of an allergic reaction, such as breathing difficulties or reddened, swollen itchy skin, particularly to the face or neck Call 999!

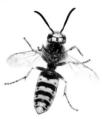

Bites

With most types of bites from animals (dogs) or humans there is the possibility of being infected from any bacteria in the saliva.

Dog bites combine deep puncture wounds where the dog grasps the skin with it's front teeth and leaves a deep hole and a laceration or scraped section of skin where the dog's bite pulls the skin.

Children tend to be bitten on the neck or face whereas, adults tend to be bitten on the hands, arms, legs or feet.

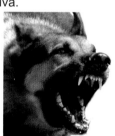

Treatment for Bites

- Wash the wound thoroughly with plenty of water.
- Pat the wound dry with a dry clean gauze.
- Cover the wound with a sterile dressing.
- If the wound is large or deep then treat the bleeding (STEP - Page 23).
- Call 999.
- If minor, advise the casualty to seek medical advice.
- Advise the casualty to seek medical advice if they are not sure if they have had a tetanus jab.
- If the bite is from another human, there is also a small risk of getting hepatitis or HIV/AIDS viruses.

1 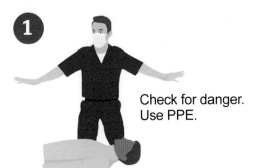 Check for danger. Use PPE.

2 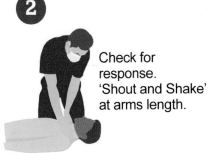 Check for response. 'Shout and Shake' at arms length.

3 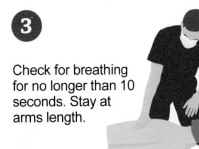 Check for breathing for no longer than 10 seconds. Stay at arms length.

STOP Do not open the airway or place your face near the casualty's mouth.

4 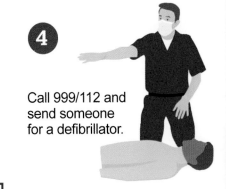 Call 999/112 and send someone for a defibrillator.

5 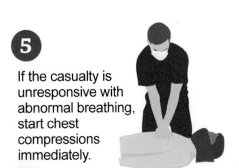 If the casualty is unresponsive with abnormal breathing, start chest compressions immediately.

STOP For protection, place a handkerchief, scarf or similar over the casualty's mouth and nose. Give continuous chest compressions, 2 per second and 5-6cm deep, pressing HARD and FAST.

6 It is completely safe to use a defibrillator on a casualty with COV 19. Switch on defibrillator and follo the instructions 'DO NOT DELAY'.